I0209950

51 Delicious Juice Recipes for Diabetics:

Naturally Control and Treat Your Diabetes Condition through Vitamin Filled Organic Ingredients

By

Joe Correa CSN

COPYRIGHT

© 2017 Live Stronger Faster Inc.

All rights reserved

Reproduction or translation of any part of this work beyond that permitted by section 107 or 108 of the 1976 United States Copyright Act without the permission of the copyright owner is unlawful.

This publication is designed to provide accurate and authoritative information in regard to the subject matter covered. It is sold with the understanding that neither the author nor the publisher is engaged in rendering medical advice. If medical advice or assistance is needed, consult with a doctor. This book is considered a guide and should not be used in any way detrimental to your health. Consult with a physician before starting this nutritional plan to make sure it's right for you.

ACKNOWLEDGEMENTS

This book is dedicated to my friends and family that have had mild or serious illnesses so that you may find a solution and make the necessary changes in your life.

51 Delicious Juice Recipes for Diabetics:

Naturally Control and Treat Your Diabetes Condition through Vitamin Filled Organic Ingredients

By

Joe Correa CSN

CONTENTS

ABOUT THE AUTHOR

After years of Research, I honestly believe in the positive effects that proper nutrition can have over the body and mind. My knowledge and experience has helped me live healthier throughout the years and which I have shared with family and friends. The more you know about eating and drinking healthier, the sooner you will want to change your life and eating habits.

Nutrition is a key part in the process of being healthy and living longer so get started today. The first step is the most important and the most significant.

INTRODUCTION

51 Delicious Juice Recipes for Diabetics: Naturally Control and Treat Your Diabetes Condition through Vitamin Filled Organic Ingredients

By Joe Correa CSN

Diabetes is one of the leading diseases in tthe modern world and preventing it is probably the best thing you can do for yourself. However, if you already have diabetes, it's not the end of the world, but it should be treated properly and kept under control.

Probably the biggest risk of diabetes is not the disease itself, but the complications that come with it. This especially goes for Type II diabetes. People know they're sick only when they feel these complications and that's exactly why its important to always keep the sugar levels in your blood in check.

The most common complications are hypoglycemia (glucose deficiency in the bloodstream) and hyperglycemia (an excess of glucose in the bloodstream). Both conditions are extremely dangerous and if not treated, can develop into ketoacidosis or hyperosmolar syndrome.

Some of the most common symptoms people feel are fatigue, confusion, or even coma. Therefore, it's always important to listen to what your body has to say and to follow a proper diet.

I have prepared this delicious and healthy collection of juices to help you fight this dangerous disease and to give you all the best nutrients a juice can possibly provide including: protein, healthy carbs, healthy fats, vitamins, minerals and amino acids. If you're like me, you might find it unusual to prepare a veggie-based juice but thats why I combined fruit to make it taste great and full of flavour. These juice recipes will give you a true nutrient bomb with amazing levels of vitamins and minerals. These amazing juice recipes have the best combinations you can possibly find out there! Did you know beet greens and brussel sprouts, found in these recipes, are proven to help normalize insulin secretion.

Be sure to try every single diabetes-friendly juice provided in this book with carefully chosen ingredients. Stay healthy and enjoy these recipes!

51 DELICIOUS JUICE RECIPES FOR DIABETICS: NATURALLY CONTROL AND TREAT YOUR DIABETES CONDITION THROUGH VITAMIN FILLED ORGANIC INGREDIENTS

1. Blueberry Juice

Ingredients:

1 cup of fresh blueberries

1 small apple

2 carrots

1 head romaine lettuce

Preparation:

Run all ingredients through a juicer. Serve cold

Nutritional information per serving: Kcal: 228, Protein: 6.14g, Carbs: 66.8g, Fats: 1.95g

2.   Pear Juice

Ingredients:

1 medium-sized pear, roughly chopped

½ cup of fresh grapes

3 large oranges

1 cup of spinach, torn

A handful of ginger, finely chopped

Preparation:

Wash and thoroughly rinse the spinach. Set aside.

Peel and section the oranges.

Run all ingredients through a juicer. Serve cold

Nutritional information per serving: Kcal: 347, Protein: 6.52g, Carbs: 108.8g, Fats: 1.27g

3.　Green Detox Juice

Ingredients:

1 cup of chopped broccoli

A bunch of fresh spinach

½ cup of coconut water, unsweetened

2 lemons

1 medium-sized orange

1 tbsp of honey, raw

few mint leaves

Preparation:

Place chopped broccoli, fresh spinach, two lemons, and orange in a juicer. Squeeze the juice and combine with unsweetened coconut water.

Add one tablespoon of raw honey and mix well.

Decorate with a couple of mint leaves and serve cold.

Nutritional information per serving: Kcal: 171, Protein: 14.8g, Carbs: 54.5g, Fats: 2.17g

4.   Berry Blast Juice

Ingredients:

1 cup of blackberries

1 cup of blueberries

1 cup of raspberries

1 cup of strawberries

¼ cup of baby spinach

½ tsp of ground ginger

Preparation:

Run the ingredients through a juicer. Sprinkle with ground ginger and serve cold.

Nutritional information per serving: Kcal: 158, Protein: 5.9g, Carbs: 56.4g, Fats: 2.3g

5.   Melon and Strawberry Juice

Ingredients:

2 cups of fresh strawberries

14 oz melon, roughly chopped

2 cups of spinach, chopped

1 medium-sized banana

½ tsp of cinnamon

1 tsp of honey, raw

Preparation:

Run strawberries, spinach, melon, and banana through a juicer.

Whisk in one teaspoon of raw honey and season with cinnamon.

Serve cold.

Nutritional information per serving: Kcal: 349, Protein: 7.6g, Carbs: 104.9g, Fats: 3.2g

6.   Strawberries smoothie

Ingredients:

2 cups of strawberries, fresh

1 cup of blueberries, fresh

½ cup of coconut water, unsweetened

½ large blood orange

1 tsp of pure coconut sugar

Preparation:

Add ingredients in a juicer, combine with coconut water and whisk in one teaspoon of pure coconut sugar.

Serve cold.

Nutritional information per serving: Kcal: 246, Protein: 4.7g, Carbs: 74.2g, Fats: 1.7g

7.   Vanilla Raspberry Juice

Ingredients:

3 cups of raspberries, fresh

½ cup of coconut water, unsweetened

½ tsp of pure vanilla extract, sugar-free

Preparation:

Place raspberries in a juicer and squeeze. Transfer to a serving glass. Add coconut water and vanilla extract.

Serve cold.

Nutritional information per serving: Kcal: 136, Protein: 4.4g, Carbs: 51.7g, Fats: 2.4g

8. Goji Juice

Ingredients:

10 oz broccoli, pre-cooked

1 cup of goji berries

1 large orange, peeled

1 large cucumber, peeled

1 tbsp of honey, raw

Preparation:

Run the ingredients through a juicer.

Whisk in honey and serve cold

Nutritional information per serving: Kcal: 193, Protein: 9.4g, Carbs: 66g, Fats: 1.7g

9.   Orange Mocha Juice

Ingredients:

½ cup of unsweetened chilled coffee

4 large oranges

1 tsp of pure vanilla extract, sugar-free

1 tsp of pure coconut sugar

Preparation:

Run oranges through a juicer.

Combine with chilled coffee and whisk in coconut sugar.

Add vanilla extract and serve cold.

Nutritional information per serving: Kcal: 292, Protein: 6.9g, Carbs: 96g, Fats: 2g

10.   Morning Carrot Juice

Ingredients:

3 large carrots

2 Alkamene apples

½ tsp of cinnamon, freshly ground

1 tbsp of honey, raw

Preparation:

Place carrots and apples in a juicer, one at the time. Squeeze the juice and transfer to a serving glass.

Add one tablespoon of honey and some cinnamon to taste.

Serve cold.

Nutritional information per serving: Kcal: 324, Protein: 3.4g, Carbs: 93g, Fats: 1.5g

11. Granny Smith Juice

Ingredients:

2 large Granny Smith apples, sliced and seeds removed

1 large grapefruit, peeled

1 tsp of honey, raw

½ tsp of ginger, freshly ground

Preparation:

Run the fruits through a juicer.

Add one teaspoon of honey and freshly ground ginger.

Serve cold.

Nutritional information per serving: Kcal: 299, Protein: 3.7g, Carbs: 88g, Fats: 1.1g

12.   Fresh Pineapple Juice

Ingredients:

1 cup of pineapple chunks

1 small apple, peeled and seeds removed

1 tsp of fresh mint leaves, finely chopped

¼ tsp of nutmeg, ground

Preparation:

Place the fruit in a juicer and squeeze.

Add ground nutmeg and mix well. Decorate with a couple of mint leaves and serve cold.

Nutritional information per serving: Kcal: 141, Protein: 1.5g, Carbs: 41.2g, Fats: 0.4g

13.   Blueberry and Banana Juice

Ingredients:

1 cup of blueberries

1 cup of blackberries

1 large banana, peeled

1 tsp of honey

½ tsp of cinnamon

Preparation:

Run the ingredients through a juicer.

Add one teaspoon of honey and cinnamon. Mix well and serve warm.

Nutritional information per serving: Kcal: 229, Protein: 4.5g, Carbs: 76.3g, Fats: 1.6g

14.   Thick Banana Juice

Ingredients:

2 large bananas

1 cup of grapes

1 tsp of pure vanilla extract, sugar-free

½ cup of coconut milk, sugar-free

Preparation:

Place bananas and grapes in a juicer. Juice and transfer to a serving glass.

Combine with coconut milk and pure vanilla extract. Serve cold.

Nutritional information per serving: Kcal: 293, Protein: 7.5g, Carbs: 77.9g, Fats: 4g

15.   Peppermint Juice

Ingredients:

3 large cucumbers, peeled

1 grapefruit, peeled

1 tsp of peppermint extract

1 tbsp of coconut sugar

Preparation:

Prepare the fruits and place in a juicer. Squeeze and add peppermint extract and coconut sugar.

Serve with some ice.

Nutritional information per serving: Kcal: 204, Protein: 7.7g, Carbs: 59g, Fats: 1.3g

16.   Flaxseed and Goji Juice

Ingredients:

1 large banana

1 cup of goji berries

1 tsp of flaxseed oil

A bunch of celery leaves

1 tbsp of honey, raw

Preparation:

Run the ingredients through a juicer. Whisk in one teaspoon of flaxseed oil and honey.

Serve with ice.

Nutritional information per serving: Kcal: 177, Protein: 6.5g, Carbs: 44.6g, Fats: 2.6g

17. Pumpkin Juice

Ingredients:

1 cup of avocado chunks

10 oz sweet pumpkin chunks

½ tsp of cinnamon, freshly ground

¼ cup of water

Preparation:

Place the fruit in a juicer and squeeze.

Combine with some water and add cinnamon.

Stir well and serve cold.

Nutritional information per serving: Kcal: 256, Protein: 5.3g, Carbs: 27.8g, Fats: 22.3g

18.   Almond Honey Juice

Ingredients:

½ cup of almond milk, sugar-free

1 tbsp of honey, raw

1 large banana, peeled

3 large red oranges, peeled

1 tbsp of fresh mint leaves, finely chopped

Preparation:

Run oranges and banana through a juicer. Combine with sugar-free almond milk and add one tablespoon of honey.

Decorate with a couple of mint leaves and serve cold.

Nutritional information per serving: Kcal: 411, Protein: 11g, Carbs: 95g, Fats: 3.1g

19.   Fresh Tomato Juice

Ingredients:

5 large tomatoes, peeled

1 cup of fresh raspberries

½ tsp of pure cherry extract, sugar-free

A couple of mint leaves

Preparation:

Run the ingredients through a juicer.

Add cherry extract and some mint to taste.

Serve immediately.

Nutritional information per serving: Kcal: 152, Protein: 9.4g, Carbs: 50g, Fats: 2.6g

20.   Greek Pomegranate Juice

Ingredients:

1 cup of pomegranate seeds

1 cup of fresh blackberries

1 large cucumber

A handful of fresh parsley

Preparation:

Place the ingredients in a juicer and squeeze.

Serve cold.

Nutritional information per serving: Kcal: 143, Protein: 7.9g, Carbs: 44.8g, Fats: 2.5g

21. Ginger and Kale Juice

Ingredients:

1 cup of kale, torn

1 cup of strawberries, fresh

½ tsp of ginger, ground

1 lemon, peeled

Preparation:

Run the ingredients through a juicer and serve cold.

Nutritional information per serving: Kcal: 120, Protein: 5.9g, Carbs: 38.6g, Fats: 1.8g

22.   Guava Juice

Ingredients:

1 whole guava

1 cup of parsnip

1 celery stalk

2 large grapefruits, peeled

Preparation:

Juice and serve cold.

Nutritional information per serving: Kcal: 279, Protein: 7.2g, Carbs: 86g, Fats: 1.7g

23. Butternut Squash Juice

Ingredients:

1 medium-sized banana, peeled

1 cup of raspberries, fresh

1 cup of butternut squash cubes

½ cup of coconut water, unsweetened

1 tsp of honey, raw

Preparation:

Run the ingredients through a juicer and combine with coconut water.

Whisk in one teaspoon of honey and serve cold.

Nutritional information per serving: Kcal: 197, Protein: 4.7g, Carbs: 68g, Fats: 1.3g

24.   Green Kiwi Juice

Ingredients:

3 large kiwis, peeled

1 cup of kale, torn

1 cup of cranberries

1 tsp of pure coconut sugar

Preparation:

Place kiwi, kale, and cranberries in a juicer. Squeeze and transfer to a serving glass.

Add one teaspoon of coconut sugar and serve cold.

Nutritional information per serving: Kcal: 153, Protein: 5.6g, Carbs: 48.4g, Fats: 1.8g

25. Summer Coconut Juice

Ingredients:

½ cup of coconut water

1 cup of pineapple chunks

1 cup of mango chunks

1 cup of guava chunks

1 tbsp of fresh mint leaves

Preparation:

Juice and sprinkle with fresh mint.

Serve cold.

Nutritional information per serving: Kcal: 187, Protein: 3.6g, Carbs: 54.2g, Fats: 1.3g

26. Mango Lime Juice

Ingredients:

1 cup of mango chunks

1 whole lime

1 cup of chard, torn

1 cup of beet greens, torn

½ cup of coconut water, unsweetened

Preparation:

Place the ingredients in a juicer and squeeze.

Combine with unsweetened coconut water and serve cold.

Nutritional information per serving: Kcal: 108, Protein: 3.8g, Carbs: 33g, Fats: 0.8g

27. Energy Juice

Ingredients:

2 large Red Delicious apples, peeled and seeds removed

1 cup of goji berries

1 cup of fresh cherries, pitted

1 cup of beets

3 large tomatoes, peeled

Preparation:

Run the ingredients through a juicer and serve immediately.

Nutritional information per serving: Kcal: 328, Protein: 9.3g, Carbs: 95g, Fats: 2.14g

28. Fresh Aronia Juice

Ingredients:

2 cups of fresh aronia

1 large banana, peeled

2 cups of spinach, torn

2 cups of beet greens, torn

Preparation:

Place the ingredients in a juicer, one at the time.

Squeeze and serve immediately.

Nutritional information per serving: Kcal: 183, Protein: 7.8g, Carbs: 63.1g, Fats: 1.2g

29.   Green Apple and Carrot Juice

Ingredients:

2 large green apples, peeled and seeds removed

3 large carrots

1 cup of parsnip slices

1 basil leaf, crushed

¼ cup of water

Preparation:

Place the ingredients in a juicer and squeeze.

Combine with water and crushed basil.

Serve cold.

Nutritional information per serving: Kcal: 332, Protein: 5.4g, Carbs: 100g, Fats: 1.6g

30.   Avocado Juice

Ingredients:

1 whole avocado, chopped

7 oz artichoke

1 medium-sized lemon, peeled

1 cup of red cabbage, shredded

1 cup of green cabbage, shredded

Preparation:

Run the ingredients through a juicer and serve immediately.

Nutritional information per serving: Kcal: 353, Protein: 12.3g, Carbs: 51g, Fats: 30g

31. Pineapple and Apricot Juice

Ingredients:

1 cup of pineapple chunks

1 cup of apricots

1 large cucumber, sliced

1 cup of fresh spinach, torn

1 whole lemon

½ cup of raw broccoli, chopped

½ cup of pure coconut water

Preparation:

Wash and prepare the ingredients.

Run through a juicer and combine with pure coconut water.

Serve immediately with ice.

Nutritional information per serving: Kcal: 218, Protein: 10g, Carbs: 64g, Fats: 1.9g

32.   Peachy Asparagus Juice

Ingredients:

1 large peach

1 cup of fresh asparagus, chopped

1 cup of collard greens

1 large grapefruit, peeled

1 cup of romaine lettuce, shredded

1 cup of fennel, sliced

Preparation:

Wash and slice the ingredients. Place in a juicer and squeeze.

Serve immediately.

Nutritional information per serving: Kcal: 187, Protein: 9.1g, Carbs: 57.9g, Fats: 1.4g

33. Plum Power Juice

Ingredients:

1 cup of plums, halved

1 cup of fresh blackberries

1 cup of turnip greens, chopped

½ tsp of ground ginger

1 tsp of coconut sugar

½ cup of water

Preparation:

Wash and slice each plum in half. Run through a juicer.

Now juice blackberries and turnip greens.

Combine in a tall serving glass. Add ground ginger and coconut sugar.

Mix well and serve.

Nutritional information per serving: Kcal: 141, Protein: 4.2g, Carbs: 40.3g, Fats: 1.4g

34.   Lemon Juice

Ingredients:

3 large lemons, peeled

1 large orange, peeled

10 oz radish

1 cup of beet greens, chopped

1 cup of watercress, chopped

1 tbsp of honey, raw

Preparation:

Peel the fruits and run through a juicer. Add radish, beet greens, and watercress. Juice and add one tablespoon of honey.

Serve cold.

Nutritional information per serving: Kcal: 147, Protein: 5.3g, Carbs: 50g, Fats: 0.8g

35.   Cherry Mint Juice

Ingredients:

2 cups of cherries, pitted

1 cup of leek, chopped

1 tbsp of fresh mint, finely chopped

1 cup of fresh cranberries

1 tbsp of honey, raw

Preparation:

Run the ingredients through a juicer.

Add one tablespoon of honey and mix well.

Serve immediately.

Nutritional information per serving: Kcal: 248, Protein: 5g, Carbs: 75.5g, Fats: 1g

36.   Leafy Ginger Juice

Ingredients:

1 cup of beet greens, chopped

1 cup of cauliflower, chopped

1 cup of fennel, sliced

1 cup of celery, chopped

1 cup of red leaf lettuce, shredded

1 cup of romaine lettuce, shredded

1 large grapefruit

½ cup of pure coconut water

1 tsp of honey

Preparation:

Wash and prepare the ingredients. Run through a juicer and add one teaspoon of honey.

Serve cold.

Nutritional information per serving: Kcal: 163, Protein: 8.3g, Carbs: 56.3g, Fats: 1.2g

37.   Sweet Mango Juice

Ingredients:

1 cup of mango, chopped

1 cup of apricots, sliced

½ cup of pure coconut water, unsweetened

1 tbsp of coconut sugar

Preparation:

Wash and slice the fruits. Juice and combine with unsweetened coconut water.

Add one tablespoon of coconut sugar.

Serve cold.

Nutritional information per serving: Kcal: 155, Protein: 3.6g, Carbs: 43g, Fats: 1.2g

38.   Apple and Peach Juice

Ingredients:

2 large golden delicious apples, peeled and seeds removed

1 large peach, chopped

1 cup of baby spinach, torn

½ cup of water

1 large carrot

½ lemon

Preparation:

Run through a juicer and serve immediately.

Nutritional information per serving: Kcal: 297, Protein: 5.5g, Carbs: 87.5g, Fats: 1.5g

39.   Fresh Ginger Juice

Ingredients:

1 large banana, peeled

1 cup of spinach, torn

2 large lemons, peeled

1 slice of ginger

1 tsp of honey

Preparation:

Place the ingredients in a juicer, one at the time.

Juice and add honey.

Serve immediately.

Nutritional information per serving: Kcal: 139, Protein: 4.5g, Carbs: 44.4g, Fats: 1.2g

40.   Papaya Juice

Ingredients:

1 cup of papaya, chopped

1 cup of goji berries

1 cup of purple cabbage, shredded

1 large blood orange, peeled

1 tsp of ginger, ground

1 tsp of honey

Preparation:

Wash and chop the ingredients. Place in a juicer, one at the time and squeeze.

Add one teaspoon of ginger and one teaspoon of honey before serving.

Nutritional information per serving: Kcal: 172, Protein: 4.3g, Carbs: 54.2g, Fats: 0.7g

41. Blueberry Juice

Ingredients:

1 cup of blueberries

2 large alkamene apples, cored and sliced

¼ cup of blackberries

1 tsp of pure mint extract, sugar-free

½ cup of water

Preparation:

Run through a juicer and serve immediately.

Nutritional information per serving: Kcal: 368, Protein: 2.5g, Carbs: 94g, Fats: 1.5g

42.   Pumpkin and Banana Juice

Ingredients:

1 cup of pumpkin cubes

1 large banana, peeled

1 large granny smith apple, peeled and cored

½ cup of pure coconut water, unsweetened

¼ tsp of nutmeg, ground

1 tbsp of coconut sugar

Preparation:

Peel and chop pumpkin. Run through a juicer.

Now add banana and apple, one at the time.

Combine with pure coconut water in a serving glass.

Add nutmeg and coconut sugar.

Serve immediately.

Nutritional information per serving: Kcal: 338, Protein: 4.6g, Carbs: 97.8g, Fats: 1.4g

43. Raspberry Lime Juice

Ingredients:

1 cup of fresh raspberries

2 limes, peeled

2 cups of raw broccoli, chopped

½ cup of coconut water, unsweetened

2 large cucumbers, peeled

1 tbsp of honey, raw

Preparation:

Run the ingredients through a juicer.

Add one tablespoon of honey and mix well.

Serve immediately.

Nutritional information per serving: Kcal: 192, Protein: 10.9g, Carbs: 56g, Fats: 2.2g

44.   Honeydew Melon Juice

Ingredients:

1 large wedge of honeydew melon

1 large radish

1 cup of chard

1 cup of asparagus

1 cup of avocado, sliced

¼ cup of pure coconut water, unsweetened

Preparation:

Wash and prepare the ingredients.

Run through a juicer and combine with unsweetened coconut water.

Serve immediately.

Nutritional information per serving: Kcal: 275, Protein: 8g, Carbs: 35.2g, Fats: 21,9g

45. Parsnip Juice

Ingredients:

1 cup of parsnip, sliced

1 large banana, peeled

1 large orange, peeled

1 cup of cauliflower, chopped

A handful of fresh mint, chopped

1 tsp of honey, raw

Preparation:

Wash, peel, and chop the ingredients. Place in a juicer and squeeze.

Transfer to a serving glass and add one teaspoon of raw honey and fresh mint.

Mix well and serve cold.

Nutritional information per serving: Kcal: 336, Protein: 8.5g, Carbs: 103g, Fats: 1.5g

46.   Mustard Green and Apple Juice

Ingredients:

1 large green apple, peeled and seeds removed

2 cups of mustard greens, chopped

1 whole leek, chopped

1 cup of Brussel sprouts

1 medium-sized zucchini, peeled

1 cup of parsnip, sliced

Preparation:

Wash and prepare the vegetables. Place in a juicer, one at the time.

Serve immediately.

Nutritional information per serving: Kcal: 284, Protein: 12.3g, Carbs: 83.7g, Fats: 2.4g

47.   Crookneck Juice

Ingredients:

1 cup of crookneck squash, sliced

1 cup of celery, chopped

1 cup of beets, sliced

1 cup of beet greens, chopped

1 cup of pomegranate seeds

1 tbsp of honey

Preparation:

Run the ingredients through a juicer.

Add one tablespoon of honey and serve immediately.

Nutritional information per serving: Kcal: 132, Protein: 6.4g, Carbs: 48.8g, Fats: 1.8g

48.   Tomato and Watercress Juice

Ingredients:

5 large tomatoes, peeled

1 cup of watercress, chopped

1 cup of turnip greens, chopped

1 cup of beets, sliced

1 tbsp of coconut sugar

½ cup of pure coconut water, unsweetened

Preparation:

Prepare the ingredients and run through a juicer.

Combine with unsweetened coconut water and add one tablespoon of coconut sugar.

Serve immediately.

Nutritional information per serving: Kcal: 212, Protein: 11.7g, Carbs: 62.7g, Fats: 2.2g

49.   Cantaloupe Juice

Ingredients:

1 cup of cantaloupe, diced

1 cup of baby spinach, torn

1 cup of cranberries

1 cup of parsley, chopped

1 medium-sized cucumber, peeled

1 tbsp of honey, raw

Preparation:

Run the ingredients through a juicer.

Add some raw honey and serve cold

Nutritional information per serving: Kcal: 197, Protein: 10.2g, Carbs: 58.3g, Fats: 2.2g

50.　Kiwi and Lime Juice

Ingredients:

1 cup of red leaf lettuce

1 cup of papaya, chopped

1 cup of cabbage, shredded

2 whole kiwis, peeled

1 whole lime, peeled

1 tsp of coconut sugar

½ cup of pure coconut water, unsweetened

Preparation:

Juice the ingredients, one at the time. Combine with coconut water and add coconut sugar.

Mix well and serve cold.

Nutritional information per serving: Kcal: 201, Protein: 7g, Carbs: 61.7g, Fats: 1.7g

51. Sweet Red Pepper Juice

Ingredients:

1 cup of red bell peppers, chopped

1 large red delicious apple, peeled and cored

2 cups of spinach, chopped

1 cup of Brussel sprouts, chopped

1 tsp of honey, raw

Preparation:

Wash and prepare the ingredients. Peel the apple and remove the seeds.

Run through a juicer and add one teaspoon of honey before serving.

Nutritional information per serving: Kcal: 196, Protein: 6.8g, Carbs: 55.6g, Fats: 1.4g

ADDITIONAL TITLES FROM THIS AUTHOR

70 Effective Meal Recipes to Prevent and Solve Being Overweight: Burn Fat Fast by Using Proper Dieting and Smart Nutrition

By

Joe Correa CSN

48 Acne Solving Meal Recipes: The Fast and Natural Path to Fixing Your Acne Problems in Less Than 10 Days!

By

Joe Correa CSN

41 Alzheimer's Preventing Meal Recipes: Reduce or Eliminate Your Alzheimer's Condition in 30 Days or Less!

By

Joe Correa CSN

70 Effective Breast Cancer Meal Recipes: Prevent and Fight Breast Cancer with Smart Nutrition and Powerful Foods

By

Joe Correa CSN

www.ingramcontent.com/pod-product-compliance
Lightning Source LLC
Chambersburg PA
CBHW051039030426
42336CB00015B/2955